MINDFUL EATING PRACTICES

A Complete Guide For Rediscover Joy In Eating And Cultivating Inner Peace, Wellness, And Connection One Meal At A Time

WALTER ZYAIRE

DISCLAIMER

The information in this book is intended only for general informational purposes; it should not be used in lieu of professional advice or medical care. Since the author is not licensed to practice therapy, the information offered should not be used in place of the expertise, judgment, or guidance of qualified mental health or medical professionals. Readers are encouraged to consult therapists, medical specialists, or other qualified authorities regarding their particular situation and needs. The publisher and author disclaim all liability for any actions or decisions taken by readers based on the information in this book. Results may vary from person to person and this book's approaches, procedures, and strategies may not be suitable in all circumstances. Considering unique situations and consulting a qualified expert are essential when choosing the right course of action. Neither the publisher nor the author recommend or guarantee the efficacy of any therapy or treatment that is indicated in this book. Because the information is based on the author's research and understanding at the time of publishing, it could not reflect the most recent developments or practices in the treatment area. The publisher and the author both disclaim all liability for the accuracy, completeness, or use of the material in this book. Readers bear full responsibility for the decisions and actions they choose in light of the information presented in this book.

TABLE OF CONTENTS

CHAPTER ONE 11

OVERVIEW OF MINDFUL EATING PRACTICES.........................11

SYNOPSIS OF INTENTIONAL CONSUMPTION 11

THE VALUE OF INTENTIONAL EATING IN EVERYDAY LIFE.................12

CHAPTER TWO 15

COMPREHENDING MINDFUL EATING 15

THE MEANING AND DEFINITION OF MINDFUL EATING 15

BACKGROUND HISTORY 16

ADVANTAGES OF INTENTIONAL EATING...........................17

CHAPTER THREE 19

THE RELATIONSHIP BETWEEN THE MIND AND BODY 19

MAKING A CONNECTION WITH SATIETY AND HUNGER....................19

IDENTIFYING EMOTIONAL EATING TRIGGERS.....................20

DURING EATING, PAYING ATTENTION TO YOUR BODY.....................21

CHAPTER FOUR 23

ACQUIRING CONSCIOUS AWARENESS 23

DEVELOPING AWARENESS OF THE PRESENT 23

HOW TO USE ALL FIVE SENSES WHEN EATING 24

WAYS TO BREATHE MINDFULLY....................................25

CHAPTER FIVE...27

BREAKING PATTERNS AND HABITS 27

RECOGNIZING UNHEALTHY FOOD HABITS.........................27

REVERSING EMOTIONAL CONSUMPTION 28

TECHNIQUES FOR ENDING MINDLESS ROUTINES 29

CHAPTER SIX 31

   CAREFUL PLANNING OF MEALS 31

      CREATING NOURISHING AND BALANCED MEALS 31

      SHOPPING WITH INTENTION 32

      MEAL PREPARATION WITH INTENTION 33

CHAPTER SEVEN 35

   CONSCIENTIOUS EATING IN VARIOUS ENVIRONMENTS 35

      EATING CONSCIOUSLY AT HOME 35

      CONSCIENTIOUS DINING IN RESTAURANTS 36

      CONSCIENTIOUS DINING DURING SOCIAL EVENTS 37

CHAPTER EIGHT 39

   CONSCIOUS EATING FOR PARTICULAR DIETS 39

      USING MINDFUL FOOD TO MANAGE YOUR WEIGHT 39

      CONSCIOUS EATING TO MANAGE SENSITIVITIES AND ALLERGIES 40

      CONSCIENTIOUS EATING FOR PARTICULAR MEDICAL CONDITIONS .. 41

CHAPTER NINE 43

   EDUCATING KIDS ON MINDFUL EATING 43

      THE VALUE OF TEACHING CHILDREN MINDFULNESS 43

      USEFUL ADVICE FOR TEACHING CHILDREN TO EAT MINDFULLY 44

      ESTABLISHING A CONSCIOUS FAMILY DINING ENVIRONMENT 45

CHAPTER TEN 47

   EXERCISE AND MOVEMENT WITH AWARENESS 47

      LINKING MINDFUL EATING TO PHYSICAL ACTIVITY 47

      INCLUDING MINDFULNESS IN EXERCISE ROUTINES 48

      FINDING JOY IN MOVEMENT 49

CHAPTER ELEVEN 51

  MAINTAINING INTENTIONAL EATING HABITS........................51

    OVERCOMING OBSTACLES 51

    ESTABLISHING A COMMUNITY OF SUPPORTIVE MINDFUL EATING...52

    INCLUDING MINDFUL EATING IN DAILY LIVING 54

ABOUT THE BOOK

The book on Mindful Eating Practices is a thorough manual created to highlight the need to develop mindfulness in our everyday food intake. The description of mindful eating in the introduction section provides context for appreciating its applicability in contemporary society. For readers, the aims and objectives provide a clear direction toward a more purposeful and healthy relationship with eating.

After defining and examining the idea, it dives into the core elements of mindful eating, giving readers a solid foundation. The historical context provides context, and a review of the advantages highlights the beneficial effects that mindful eating can have on general health.

The mind-body link is the subject, which highlights the significance of identifying emotional triggers, detecting hunger and fullness indicators, and being aware of bodily feelings throughout meals. In establishing a holistic approach, this part recognizes the connection between mental and physical factors in eating habits.

The reader is guided through the process of growing mindful awareness through the use of practical strategies like activating the senses, fostering present-moment awareness, and adding mindful breathing techniques. The goal of these exercises is to improve the reader's capacity for mindful and present-minded eating.

The book shifts to techniques for ending habits and patterns, assisting readers in recognizing and overcoming bad eating behaviors as well as dealing with emotional eating. The topic of mindful meal planning is expanded upon, where the emphasis is on preparing wholesome, well-balanced meals, buying with awareness, and preparing meals with purpose.

The application of mindful eating in various contexts and for particular diets is covered, giving readers useful advice on how to include mindfulness at home, in restaurants, or when managing particular medical problems. In addition to providing helpful advice for setting up a mindful dining environment in the home, it discusses the significance of teaching mindfulness to young readers.

The focus of the book widens in the following chapters, which include the discussion of the link between mindful eating and exercise advice on maintaining mindful eating habits. These sections encourage readers to incorporate mindfulness into their daily lives by providing a comprehensive approach to well-being.

This book is an invaluable tool for anyone who wants to develop a mindful eating style. It provides helpful advice, methods, and a thorough grasp of how these practices affect mental, physical, and emotional health.

CHAPTER ONE

OVERVIEW OF MINDFUL EATING PRACTICES

SYNOPSIS OF INTENTIONAL CONSUMPTION

A comprehensive approach to eating that emphasizes a deep connection between the mind and body during meals, mindful eating goes beyond the act of merely consuming food. Its foundation lies in the antiquated Buddhist idea of mindfulness, which exhorts people to eat with complete awareness and present mindfulness. In contrast to mindlessly ingesting food or racing through meals, mindful eating promotes an intentional and thoughtful approach to the complete food consumption process.

By doing this, people can learn to appreciate the sensory qualities of food, savor every bite, and become more conscious of their own hunger and fullness indicators.

Mindful eating is much more than just calculating calories or following a rigid diet. It encourages a more perceptive and intuitive connection with food, emphasizing the quality of the meal rather than strict dietary guidelines.

People can develop a better knowledge of their bodies' requirements, a better relationship with food, and possibly even more enjoyment from their meals by introducing mindfulness into their eating patterns.

THE VALUE OF INTENTIONAL EATING IN EVERYDAY LIFE

The value of mindful eating is becoming more and more apparent in daily life as societies struggle with issues like stress, fast-paced lifestyles, and the overabundance of processed meals.

The fast-paced and preoccupied nature of modern life frequently encourages people to eat quickly while multitasking or in front of computers. Eating hurriedly can cause dissociation from the sensory experience of food, which can make it challenging to appropriately identify sensations of fullness and hunger.

A counterpoint to these tendencies is provided by mindful eating, which encourages people to slow down and interact more intentionally with their meals.

A more satisfying and nourishing eating experience can be achieved by encouraging mindfulness during the meal. This will increase a person's awareness of the tastes, textures, and scents of their food.

Furthermore, mindful eating has been linked to several health advantages, such as better weight management, better digestion, and a lower chance of developing problematic eating habits like binge eating or emotional eating.

Essentially, mindful eating promotes a more harmonic and balanced relationship between the mind and the act of feeding oneself by encouraging people to approach meals with curiosity and mindfulness.

We discover a road towards a more thoughtful and satisfying manner of feeding our bodies as we delve into the subtleties of mindful eating and examine its implications in day-to-day life.

CHAPTER TWO

COMPREHENDING MINDFUL EATING

THE MEANING AND DEFINITION OF MINDFUL EATING

The goal of mindful eating is to cultivate a heightened awareness and presence throughout the entire eating experience. It is a holistic approach to food consumption. In essence, mindful eating involves cultivating a non-judgmental awareness of one's thoughts and feelings around food, being present in the moment, and paying careful attention to the sensory components of eating. This technique is based on mindfulness meditation, which promotes an inactive awareness of the here and now. When it comes to eating, it refers to taking pleasure in every bite, paying attention to signals of hunger and fullness, and choosing carefully what and how much to eat.

There is more to attentive eating than just chewing and swallowing. It includes every step of the process, including meal preparation and consumption as well as meal planning and food selection. Understanding how our relationship with food is influenced by both physical and emotional aspects is a key component of mindful eating. By adopting this strategy, people can overcome automatic and habitual eating habits and develop a more meaningful and fulfilling relationship with the act of eating.

BACKGROUND HISTORY

Though the phrase "mindful eating" has become more popular recently, its origins are in antiquated contemplative traditions like mindfulness and Zen Buddhism. These customs place a strong emphasis on living in the present and giving every task—eating included—your whole attention. The Mindfulness-Based Stress Reduction (MBSR) program was developed by Jon Kabat-Zinn in the late 1970s, and it is credited with bringing mindful eating into Western culture today. The groundwork for utilizing mindfulness concepts, especially those about eating, to enhance general well-being and lessen stress was established by Kabat-Zinn's work.

Dr. Jan Chozen Bays and Dr. Lilian Cheung have been instrumental in bringing mindful eating to a wider audience. In "Savor: Mindful Eating, Mindful Life," Dr. Cheung and Dr. Bays provide useful activities and practical insights to assist people in cultivating a more conscious connection with food.

With time, mindful eating has become a common practice and has been included in several therapeutic and wellness initiatives.

ADVANTAGES OF INTENTIONAL EATING

Eating mindfully has numerous psychological, emotional, and physical advantages. Improving digestion and encouraging healthier eating habits are two of the main benefits. People can better control their food intake and maintain a more nutritious and well-balanced diet by paying close attention to their hunger and fullness cues.

The exercise also fosters a greater appreciation for food's sensory qualities, which raises the pleasure of meals in general.

By lowering emotional and impulsive eating, mindful eating can, from a psychological standpoint, assist people in creating a better relationship with food. People can recognize and deal with emotional triggers that might lead to harmful eating patterns by being mindful and nonjudgmental when eating. This increased consciousness encourages a good attitude toward eating by giving one a sense of empowerment and control over their decisions.

However, mindful eating has advantages that go beyond the dinner table. Studies indicate that engaging in mindful eating practices can help lower stress levels and enhance mental health in general. A mindful eating practice can improve people's quality of life in general and have a positive knock-on effect on many facets of happiness and health.

CHAPTER THREE

THE RELATIONSHIP BETWEEN THE MIND AND BODY

MAKING A CONNECTION WITH SATIETY AND HUNGER

Recognizing and acting upon our bodies' signals of hunger and fullness is essential to understanding the mind-body connection. This relationship explores a deeper comprehension of the body's signals and goes beyond the act of eating. In addition to being a bodily experience, hunger is also impacted by psychological variables.

Developing a connection with hunger requires being aware of the body's subtle cues, such as growling in the stomach, a sense of emptiness, or a decrease in energy. Acknowledging these indicators enables people to develop a more intuitive connection with their bodies, encouraging a more attentive and health-conscious eating style.

Similar to this, a key component of the mind-body relationship is realizing fullness. It necessitates being aware of the body's indications of fulfillment and satisfaction. Savoring each meal and giving the brain time to detect fullness are two benefits of mindful eating. People can have a more harmonious connection with food and enhance their general well-being by learning to connect with their feelings of hunger and fullness.

IDENTIFYING EMOTIONAL EATING TRIGGERS

The complex link between eating habits and emotions is another example of the mind-body connection. Emotional stressors frequently cause people to turn to food for comfort or diversion, resulting in a complicated interaction between the mind and body. One of the most important first steps toward creating a more positive relationship between mental health and physical sustenance is recognizing these emotional triggers.

Emotional eating can occur as a reaction to happiness, boredom, stress, or despair. To identify these triggers, it becomes imperative to cultivate emotional intelligence and self-awareness. Understanding the underlying emotions that motivate particular eating behaviors can be greatly aided by practicing mindfulness exercises like journaling and meditation. People can develop a more balanced and thoughtful relationship with food and end the pattern of using food as a coping mechanism for emotional discomfort by identifying and resolving emotional triggers.

DURING EATING, PAYING ATTENTION TO YOUR BODY SENSATIONS

A key component of the mind-body connection that encourages mindful eating is paying attention to one's bodily experiences while eating. This entails using all of your senses, paying attention to the textures, flavors, and scents of the food, and being completely present while you eat.

By doing this, people can develop a stronger bond between their body and mind by becoming more conscious of the eating experience.

Noticing the cues of fullness and contentment as they arise is another aspect of tuning into physical feelings. The body may communicate with the brain to let it know when it has had enough food by eating slowly and relishing every bite. This conscious eating method promotes a healthier relationship with food in addition to improved digestion.

A holistic approach that acknowledges the complex interactions between mental and physical well-being involves the mind-body link about hunger and fullness, emotional triggers for eating, and tuning into bodily sensations when eating. A more harmonious and balanced relationship with food can result from practicing mindfulness in these areas, which can enhance general health and well-being.

CHAPTER FOUR

ACQUIRING CONSCIOUS AWARENESS

DEVELOPING AWARENESS OF THE PRESENT

Cultivating a heightened sense of present-moment awareness, or being completely involved and attentive to the current experience without passing judgment, is a necessary step towards developing mindful awareness. It takes deliberate effort to turn one's attention from worries about the past or the future to how the present is developing.

By encouraging people to notice their feelings, ideas, and physical experiences as they emerge, this technique helps people develop a strong sense of present-moment awareness.

Being in the present moment means recognizing the past and future without becoming caught up in their emotional hold. It does not mean rejecting plans for the future or neglecting the past. It places a strong emphasis on observing ideas and feelings without passing judgment, which enables people to react to circumstances more deftly. People can improve their comprehension of their responses and foster emotional stability and inner serenity by practicing this awareness.

HOW TO USE ALL FIVE SENSES WHEN EATING

By encouraging people to use all five senses when eating, mindful eating can turn a routine activity into a very satisfying sensory encounter. This method emphasizes a deliberate and aware relationship with every bite, as opposed to mindlessly swallowing food. People's appreciation of the culinary experience is enhanced when they focus on the flavors, textures, colors, scents, and sounds of the food.

Using all five senses when eating fosters a closer relationship with the sustenance that food provides. It makes it possible for people to slow down and cultivate appreciation for the food and the finer points of the dish.

A healthy and intuitive relationship with food can be fostered by this mindful approach, which can help people become more aware of their bodies' signals of hunger and fullness and develop healthier eating habits.

WAYS TO BREATHE MINDFULLY

The first step toward cultivating attentive awareness is mindful breathing. It entails using the breath as an anchor to the present moment by paying close attention to it.

Amid the everyday chaos, people can establish a place for calmness and serenity by paying close attention to their breaths as they come and go. This method is a useful tool for developing awareness because it is easily obtainable and portable.

There are many different mindful breathing exercises available, from basic diaphragmatic breathing to more complex methods like box breathing or alternate nostril breathing.

These methods assist people in being more resilient to stressors in addition to fostering calm. Consistently engaging in mindful breathing exercises strengthens the link between the mind and body, cultivating a sense of peace and balance that permeates all facets of life.

CHAPTER FIVE

BREAKING PATTERNS AND HABITS

RECOGNIZING UNHEALTHY FOOD HABITS

It is essential to comprehend and recognize bad eating habits to start a transforming path towards improved health. Unhealthy eating patterns can take many different forms, including dependence on processed and nutrient-poor meals, emotional eating, and mindless snacking. Identifying these patterns entails being more conscious of one's food choices, keeping an eye out for situations that can prompt unhealthy eating, and realizing how these actions affect one's general well-being.

To identify unhealthy patterns, it is crucial to keep an eye on the kinds of food eaten, how often meals are taken, and the environment in which eating occurs. People who possess this self-awareness can identify whether they tend to skip meals, overindulge in sugary snacks, or participate in other unhealthy eating practices. Breaking free from the unhealthy eating cycle requires determining the underlying causes of these tendencies, be they stress, boredom, or emotional triggers.

REVERSING EMOTIONAL CONSUMPTION

One prevalent and difficult component of bad eating behaviors that frequently calls for a more thorough understanding and an all-encompassing strategy to overcome is emotional eating. Using food as a coping method for stress, depression, or other emotional triggers is known as emotional eating. It takes the development of alternate techniques for efficient emotion management to break this cycle. Gaining emotional intelligence and mindfulness can help people become more aware of their emotions, which will make it simpler to meet emotional demands without turning to food as a crutch.

Establishing a nurturing atmosphere is also essential to overcoming emotional eating.

This entails creating a network of people who can support you emotionally, participating in happy and fulfilling activities, and getting help from a professional if necessary. One of the most important skills in ending the emotional eating cycle is being able to distinguish between actual and emotional hunger. People can progressively stop using food as a coping technique for their emotions by cultivating emotional resilience and stronger coping processes.

TECHNIQUES FOR ENDING MINDLESS ROUTINES

Whether they are related to food or other areas of life, mindless habits are frequently the result of habitual behaviors and routines. It takes a combination of self-awareness, deliberate decision-making, and persistent effort to break these behaviors. By practicing mindfulness practices like focused attention and conscious breathing, people can disrupt the automatic pattern of thoughtless habits and become more cognizant of what they are doing.

Breaking mindless habits can also be effectively achieved by setting clear and attainable goals. By setting specific goals, people can chart a course for transformation and track their advancement over time. Gradually altering routines and surroundings can also upset established patterns, which facilitate the replacement of thoughtless habits with deliberate, health-promoting actions.

Additionally, asking friends, family, or a mentor for help can be a great way to get accountability and support when trying to stop thoughtless habits. Having a robust support network makes it easier to foster an environment that is inspiring and conducive to long-term transformation. Acknowledging minor triumphs during the journey strengthens the resolve to overcome thoughtless routines, promoting a feeling of empowerment and success. In the end, self-awareness, deliberate effort, and continued support are necessary to overcome mindless patterns and create a path toward long-lasting, beneficial change.

CHAPTER SIX

CAREFUL PLANNING OF MEALS

CREATING NOURISHING AND BALANCED MEALS

Mindful meal planning entails the purposeful and careful preparation of nourishing and balanced meals that promote general well-being. This process must take into account the nutritional worth of every ingredient and guarantee that the proportions of proteins, carbs, fats, vitamins, and minerals are balanced. A well-proportioned meal meets the body's energy requirements and improves cognitive performance in addition to providing nourishment.

Lean proteins, whole grains, healthy fats, and a range of vibrant fruits and vegetables are all necessary for achieving balance. In addition to offering a range of nutrients, this diversity gives meals a sensory element that enhances their enjoyment. A thoughtful meal plan transcends simple nutrition and becomes a comprehensive strategy for promoting health and energy by recognizing the nutritional synergies between various food groups.

SHOPPING WITH INTENTION

Conscious and intentional shopping behaviors are the first step in mindful meal planning at the grocery store. It entails selecting ingredients based on knowledge of their quality and source. Making fresh, locally grown produce and whole foods a priority benefits one's health as well as the livelihoods of nearby farmers and sustainable farming methods. Conscientious consumers read labels, choose products that are high in nutrients and low in processing, and stay away from products that have a lot of additives or preservatives.

Making a thorough grocery list based on the week's meal plan in advance is a crucial part of mindful shopping. This keeps impulse buys at bay and guarantees that the components needed for wholesome, well-balanced meals are always in stock.

Furthermore, observing the fresh produce's hues, textures, and scents while shopping adds a sensory element to the process and strengthens the link between nutrition and well-being.

Intentional meal preparation entails approaching the entire cooking process with mindfulness. Before going into the kitchen, it is important to have an optimistic and determined attitude. Simple rituals like pausing to breathe deeply and expressing gratitude for the ingredients being used might help achieve this. While preparing meals, practicing mindfulness not only improves the taste experience but also adds to the overall contentment and joy that comes from the food.

People may be present and enjoy the textures, colors, and scents of the ingredients when they take the time to carefully cut, slice, and cook. A mindful approach to meal preparation also involves controlling portion sizes, abstaining from excess, and respecting your body's natural hunger and satiety cues. This deliberate technique carries over to the final dish's presentation, resulting in an aesthetically pleasing and delicious meal that improves the dining experience even more.

Conscious meal planning includes meal preparation with intention, mindful buying, and the development of nutritious and well-balanced meals. By incorporating these practices into our daily lives, we promote a more holistic approach to nutrition and health by fostering not only physical well-being but also a deeper connection to the food we eat.

CHAPTER SEVEN

CONSCIENTIOUS EATING IN VARIOUS ENVIRONMENTS

EATING CONSCIOUSLY AT HOME

The discipline of applying awareness and intention to the entire eating experience is fundamental to mindful eating at home. To do this, one must develop a close relationship with the food, the eating process, and the body's cues. People can establish an atmosphere that supports mindful eating in their homes.

This could entail minimizing outside distractions like television or electrical devices, creating a cozy and serene environment, and giving each bite your whole focus.

Making thoughtful decisions when preparing and organizing meals is just as important as actually eating when eating mindfully at home. This entails choosing complete, nutrient-dense dishes and enjoying the cooking process.

From choosing ingredients to enjoying the finished dish, people can cultivate a mindful relationship with food in the comforts of their own homes by being present throughout the entire food experience.

CONSCIENTIOUS DINING IN RESTAURANTS

The social aspect of dining out and the distractions from outside stimuli can make mindful eating in a restaurant setting particularly difficult. Notwithstanding these obstacles, people can practice mindfulness by choosing carefully and giving their whole attention to the meal.

This entails enjoying flavors, being mindful of portion proportions, and appreciating the work that goes into making each dish.

It's imperative to fight the urge to eat quickly when at a restaurant. Eating mindfully involves taking breaks between bites, having meaningful discussions, and enjoying the restaurant's atmosphere. Furthermore, choosing menu items thoughtfully by individual health preferences and goals promotes awareness and control in a dining environment.

CONSCIENTIOUS DINING DURING SOCIAL EVENTS

Food is a common topic of conversation during social events, which offers both advantages and disadvantages for mindful eating. Managing buffet-style gatherings or parties necessitates paying close attention to signs of hunger and fullness. It entails paying attention to your body's cues and making deliberate decisions about what and how much to eat.

Being conscious in social situations includes striking a balance between chatting and enjoying your meal. A holistic mindful experience involves not only focusing on the act of eating but also being present with those around you.

Furthermore, valuing each person's dietary preferences and encouraging a nonjudgmental outlook on one's own and other people's food choices improves people's general sense of well-being when they eat in social settings.

Mindful eating is a habit that adapts to the particular opportunities and problems that each setting brings. A happier and better connection with food can result from practicing mindfulness during meals, whether at home, at restaurants, or in social settings.

CHAPTER EIGHT

CONSCIOUS EATING FOR PARTICULAR DIETS

USING MINDFUL FOOD TO MANAGE YOUR WEIGHT

A comprehensive strategy for feeding the body is mindful eating, which can be especially helpful for people trying to control their weight. Those who practice mindful eating are encouraged to develop a keen awareness of their eating patterns rather than following tight regimens. This entails being aware of indicators related to hunger and fullness, enjoying every bite, and understanding the emotional components of eating. People can have a healthier connection with eating and potentially achieve more lasting weight management by cultivating a mindful approach to food.

Differentiating between emotional and physical hunger is crucial when using mindful eating to manage weight.

By being able to identify true bodily hunger, mindful eaters are better able to meet their body's nutritional needs. People who are aware of their bodies' cues might avoid overindulging and emotional eating episodes by deliberately choosing when and what to eat. In the end, this increased awareness can help achieve weight management objectives by promoting better portion control and a better comprehension of the body's satiety cues.

CONSCIOUS EATING TO MANAGE SENSITIVITIES AND ALLERGIES

Mindful eating becomes even more important for people who have allergies or sensitivity. In this case, mindful eating is paying close attention to the components and any potential allergies in each bite in addition to being mindful of the moment during food consumption. It necessitates paying more attention to food labels, comprehending cooking techniques, and being watchful for cross-contamination hazards.

To better understand how different foods affect their bodies, mindful eaters with allergies and sensitivities learn to approach their meals with a spirit of inquiry and curiosity. By keeping an eye out for any negative reactions or sensitivities and recording them, people are better equipped to make decisions that put their health and well-being first.

In addition, mindfulness training helps lessen food-related anxiety, promoting a healthier relationship with food despite the difficulties caused by allergies or sensitivities.

CONSCIENTIOUS EATING FOR PARTICULAR MEDICAL CONDITIONS

It is possible to modify mindful eating to meet the particular nutritional requirements linked to particular medical problems. People with diabetes, heart problems, or digestive diseases can all benefit from changing the way they think about eating to include mindfulness.

This entails being aware of the dietary needs related to their health condition, selecting foods carefully, and continuing to be mindful of the effects of various foods on their overall well-being.

When it comes to particular medical issues, mindful eating frequently entails working with nutritionists or dietitians to customize meals to meet individual needs. Depending on the health issue, it could also entail keeping an eye on blood sugar levels, considering food glycemic index, or limiting sodium consumption. People can cultivate a sense of empowerment and actively engage in their overall health and wellness journey by incorporating mindfulness into food management.

CHAPTER NINE

EDUCATING KIDS ON MINDFUL EATING

THE VALUE OF TEACHING CHILDREN MINDFULNESS

It is crucial to teach children mindfulness, particularly when it comes to eating, to promote their general well-being and help them form a positive relationship with food. Children who practice mindful eating are more likely to interact with their senses, live in the present, and become more conscious of their eating patterns. Early instillation of these behaviors by parents and educators lays the groundwork for a pleasant and attentive relationship with food that benefits one's physical and mental well-being.

The development of awareness is a vital component of teaching kids to eat mindfully. Children are frequently exposed to distractions during meals, such as technological gadgets or hectic schedules, in today's fast-paced society.

They are prompted by mindfulness to slow down, appreciate each bite, and pay attention to the flavors, textures, and colors of their meal. This increased consciousness fosters a stronger bond between them and the nutritive content of the food they eat, in addition to improving their sensory experience.

 Teaching kids to identify and act upon their hunger and fullness cues is essential, in addition to raising awareness. Children who practice mindful eating are better able to distinguish between physical and emotional hunger by learning to listen to their bodies. Children who are aware of these signs can have a healthy connection with food and make decisions based more on what their bodies need than on what other people think.

USEFUL ADVICE FOR TEACHING CHILDREN TO EAT MINDFULLY

Incorporating easy exercises and activities into every day routines is one of the practical suggestions for educating youngsters about mindful eating. When a child is about to eat, for instance, parents can encourage "mindful moments" where the youngster takes a few deep breaths and expresses thanks for the food in front of them. Children who help prepare meals also develop a stronger bond with the food and become more aware of its nutritional value and place of origin.

ESTABLISHING A CONSCIOUS FAMILY DINING ENVIRONMENT

For these habits to be perpetuated, it is essential to establish a mindful eating environment in the family. Taking time to appreciate the food and each other's company during family dinners helps facilitate shared awareness. Creating a practice of switching off electronics at mealtimes and encouraging candid communication are two more ways to help create a family environment that values mindful eating.

In addition, parents are extremely important as role models for their kids. Children's conduct can be greatly influenced by exhibiting attentive eating behaviors themselves, such as savoring every piece and eating without interruptions. Family conversations about the value of mindful eating and how it improves general health can serve to further solidify these ideas and foster a commitment to a mindful eating style.

Teaching kids to be mindful while they eat is an important investment in their well-being. Parents and teachers may help children build a healthy and long-lasting connection with food by raising awareness, teaching them how to recognize and respond to hunger and fullness cues, and modeling mindful eating in the home. This method fosters a mindful mindset that may be applied to many aspects of their lives in addition to promoting physical health.

CHAPTER TEN

EXERCISE AND MOVEMENT WITH AWARENESS

LINKING MINDFUL EATING TO PHYSICAL ACTIVITY

A comprehensive approach to well-being includes both mindful eating and physical activity. The awareness and presence that people bring to their daily routines is what connects these two principles. Eating mindfully teaches people to enjoy every meal, pay attention to their body's signals of hunger and fullness, and enjoy the sensory experience of eating. When one applies this mindfulness to physical exercise, movement, and nutrition come into play in harmony.

When exercising mindfully, one must be present in the moment, experience all of the sensations, and pay attention to how one's body moves. A stronger bond between the mental and physical selves can be fostered by expanding this awareness to include how the body reacts to physical activity. Through the integration of mindful eating with physical activity, people cultivate a holistic awareness of their bodies, ultimately improving their general health and well-being.

INCLUDING MINDFULNESS IN EXERCISE ROUTINES

Mindfulness is a potent tool that may be used to change boring workouts into enjoyable and meaningful experiences. People can develop a mind-body connection that extends beyond physical exertion by becoming cognizant of their movements instead of just performing the motions mechanically. When exercising, mindfulness entails paying attention to your breath, how your muscles feel, and how it feels to be fully present in the moment.

Exercise-related mindfulness helps people become more aware of their bodies, which lowers the risk of injury and encourages a more sustainable and balanced approach to fitness.

As people intentionally move to remove tension and stress, mindful exercise also promotes mental clarity. Exercise regimens that include mindfulness can be transformed into meditation practices that benefit the body and mind, whether the exercise is yoga, running, or weightlifting.

FINDING JOY IN MOVEMENT

This concept goes beyond the idea that working out should be seen as a chore or a way to get somewhere. On the contrary, it motivates people to find fulfillment and joy in moving their bodies. This method is consistent with mindful movement, stressing the value of enjoying the trip and being present rather than obsessing about objectives or results.

Joy in motion can take many different forms, ranging from the sheer delight of a stroll through the outdoors to the thrilling experience of unrestricted dance. People who find joy in moving are more likely to stick to a regular and long-lasting fitness regimen.

In addition to the physical advantages of regular exercise, this positive correlation with physical activity promotes mental and emotional health, which adds to overall well-being.

A holistic approach to well-being is facilitated by the combination of mindful eating with physical activity, the introduction of mindfulness into exercise regimens, and the emphasis on finding joy in movement. People can develop a stronger bond with their bodies and support a sustainable and balanced route to health and happiness by encouraging awareness, presence, and enjoyment in both eating and moving.

CHAPTER ELEVEN

MAINTAINING INTENTIONAL EATING HABITS

OVERCOMING OBSTACLES

Despite being a transformational and liberating practice, mindful eating is not without its difficulties. The fast-paced nature of modern living is one frequent barrier that frequently encourages careless eating habits. Meals may be hurried due to the demands of work, family, and other obligations, which makes it challenging to fully enjoy and savor each bite. Creating space for mindful eating in the middle of a busy schedule requires making a conscious effort to prioritize and set aside time for meals to overcome this difficulty.

The ubiquity of outside temptations like television, smart phones, and other electronics presents another challenge. Distractions like these can take focus away from the sensory experience of eating, which can result in overindulgence and decreased satisfaction. Setting deliberate limits and establishing tech-free areas during meals is necessary to overcome this obstacle and foster conscious awareness of the eating process.

Furthermore, one's relationship with food might be impacted by cultural influences and societal pressures. Mindless overeating is encouraged by social events, commercials, and societal standards that prioritize quantity over quality.

Developing self-awareness, comprehending one's triggers, and making deliberate decisions in line with mindful eating concepts are necessary to overcome this obstacle. It is essential to cultivate resistance despite outside stimuli to continue eating mindfully.

ESTABLISHING A COMMUNITY OF SUPPORTIVE MINDFUL EATING

This practice can be made much more sustainable by establishing a community of supportive mindful eaters.

A community of people with similar ideals and experiences can offer support and compassion along the sometimes difficult road toward mindful eating. Creating a small support group with friends or family, taking part in online forums, or joining local mindfulness or wellness groups are just a few methods to foster this community.

Mutual support and a sense of camaraderie are fostered within the group through sharing personal problems and accomplishments. A good and caring environment is created by having candid discussions regarding mindful eating techniques, sharing advice, and acknowledging successes. Furthermore, participating in group meditation sessions or mindfulness workshops can enhance community ties and increase personal dedication to the mindful eating path.

Moreover, it can be advantageous to find accountability partners in the community. A feeling of accountability and drive is provided by frequent check-ins and agreed-upon objectives. Overcoming obstacles and upholding a long-term commitment to mindful eating can be greatly aided by the combined energy of a caring mindful eating community.

INCLUDING MINDFUL EATING IN DAILY LIVING

To maintain mindful eating habits, it is crucial to incorporate them easily into daily living. Rather than being seen as a stand-alone activity, mindful eating ought to integrate organically and intuitively into everyday activities. The first step in this integration is to create a conscious atmosphere, which includes designating a specific area for meals, reducing outside distractions, and selecting healthful and aesthetically pleasing foods.

Another important component is to include mindfulness when preparing meals. The act of cooking with gratitude and intention improves the mindful eating experience in its entirety. Wholesome, fresh food selection and quantity control are important components of a comprehensive mindful nutrition strategy.

Beyond the dinner table, mindful eating includes grocery shopping and being conscious of the foods you choose in different situations. Having a mindful attitude toward food entails learning to appreciate the origins of products, comprehending nutritional information, and making deliberate decisions that support one's health.

Furthermore, long-term sustainability depends on engaging in mindfulness practices during stressful or emotional eating episodes. Healthy eating habits include identifying emotional triggers, practicing mindful breathing, and selecting healthy coping mechanisms. A long-lasting and sustained commitment to mindful eating is fostered by the progressive incorporation of these practices into daily life, which in turn promotes general well-being and mindful living.